My First Book of Emotions for Toddlers

To Carlton, Galen, Dante, Celeste, and Sebastian, my amazing family. Thank you for teaching me about emotions. I love you all.

For general information on our other products and services or to obtain technical support, please contact our Customer Care Department within the United States at (866) 744-2665, or outside the United States at (510) 253-0500.

Rockridge Press publishes its books in a variety of electronic and print formats. Some content that appears in print may not be available in electronic books, and vice versa.

TRADEMARKS: Rockridge Press and the Rockridge Press logo are trademarks or registered trademarks of Callisto Media Inc. and/or its affiliates, in the United States and other countries, and may not be used without written permission. All other trademarks are the property of their respective owners. Rockridge Press is not associated with any product or vendor mentioned in this book.

Interior and Cover Designer: Lisa Forde
Art Producer: Samantha Ulban
Editor: Mary Colgan
Production Editor: Nora Milman
Production Manager: David Zapanta

Illustrations © 2022 April Hartmann.
Author photo courtesy of Cristina Quillez Diaz.

Paperback ISBN: 978-1-68539-074-7
eBook ISBN: 978-1-68539-403-5
R0

Printed in Canada

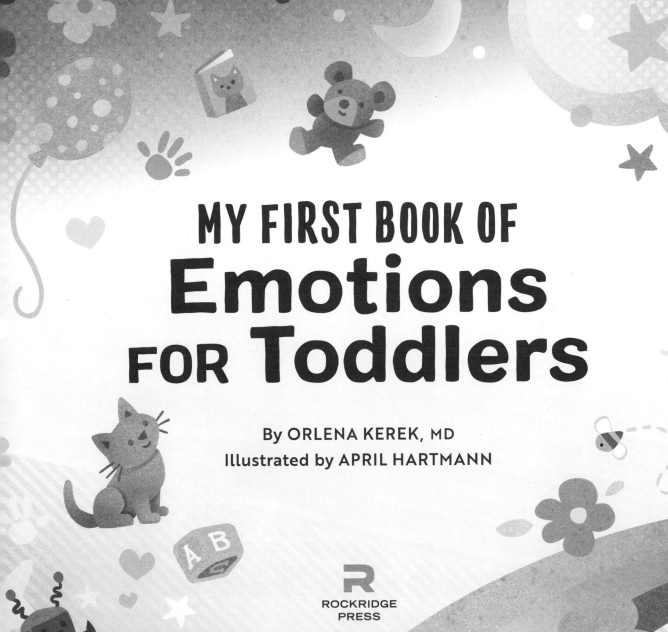

MY FIRST BOOK OF
Emotions
FOR Toddlers

By ORLENA KEREK, MD

Illustrated by APRIL HARTMANN

ROCKRIDGE PRESS

How are you feeling?

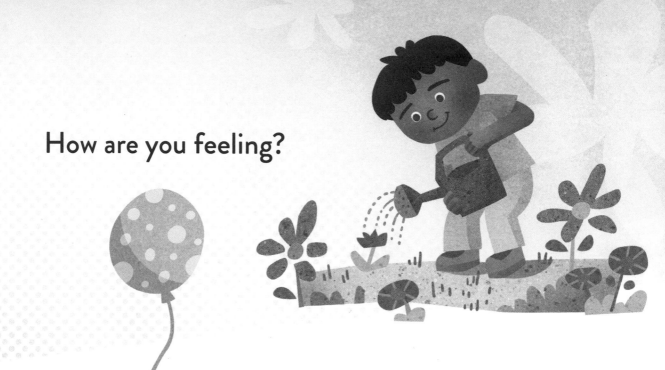

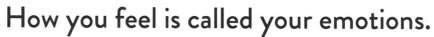

How you feel is called your emotions.

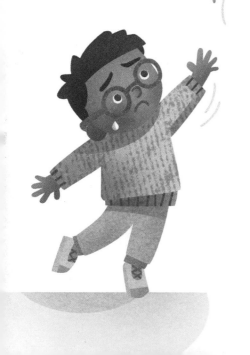

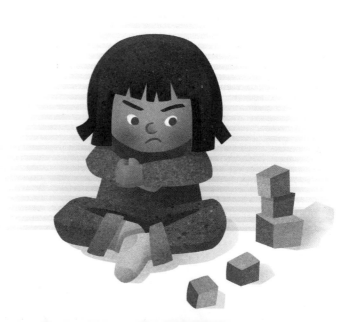

Everyone has emotions.

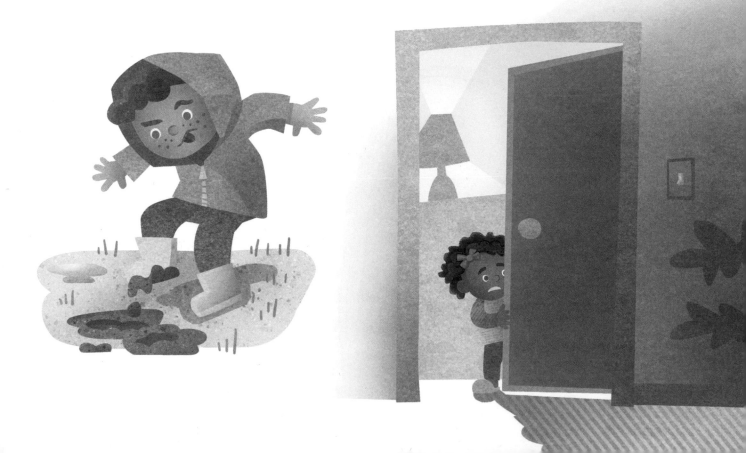

Emotions can be big or small.
They can make you laugh
or cry or jump or shout.

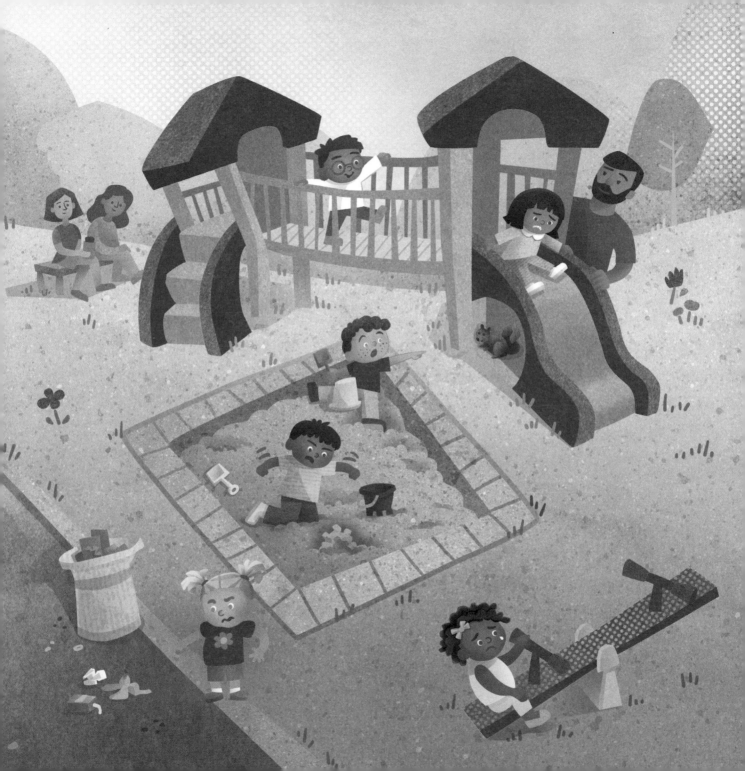

Telling people about your emotions
lets them know how you feel.

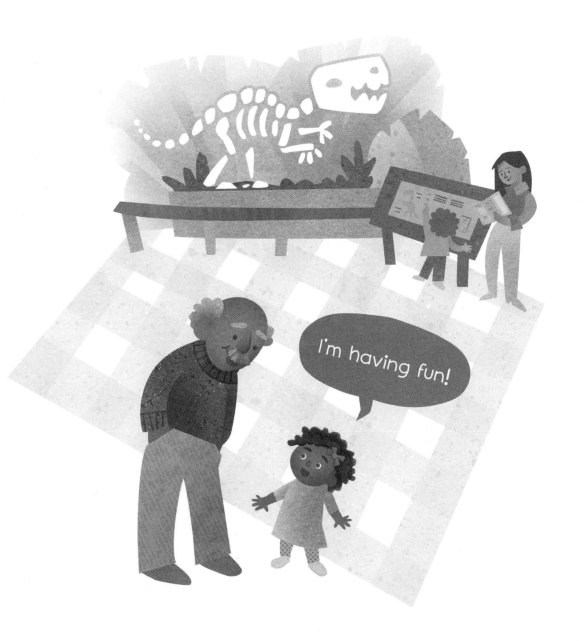

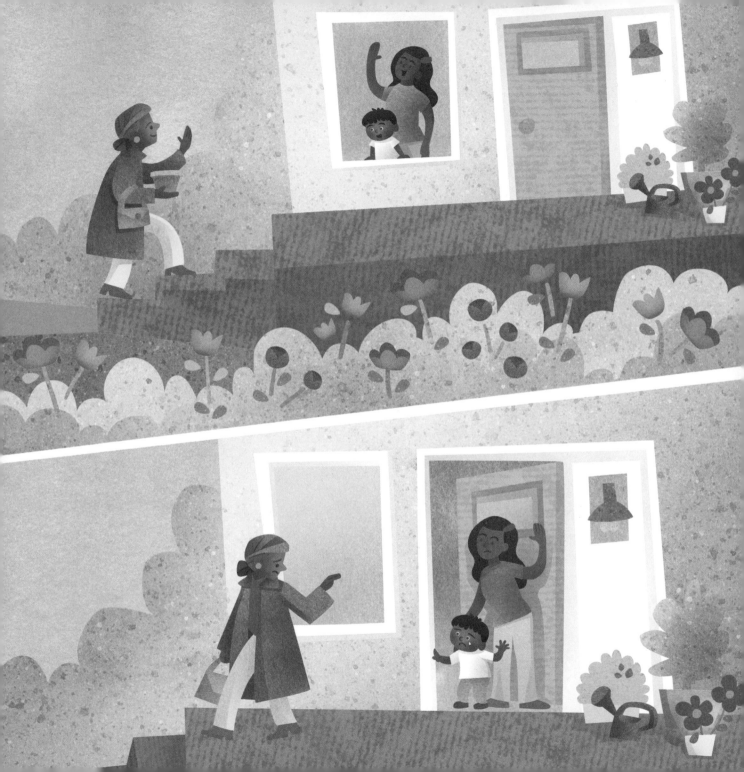

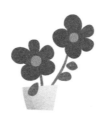

When good or bad things happen,
your body feels emotions.

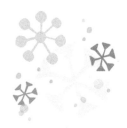

When you are happy,
your body feels light and warm. You might
smile, clap, and say, "Hooray!"
What makes you happy?

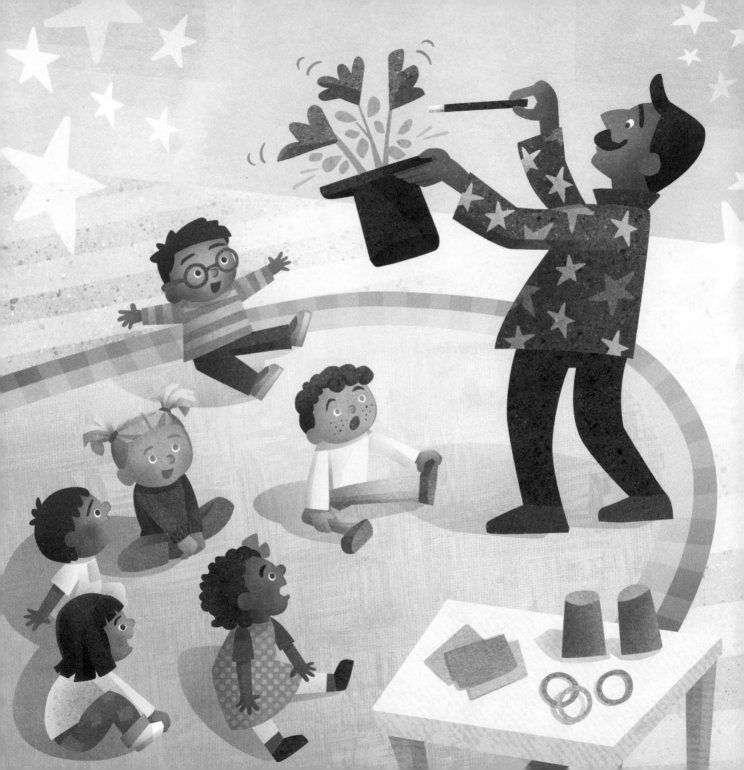

You feel surprised when something
happens that you didn't expect.
You might gasp, open your eyes wide,
and say, "Oh!"

What surprises you?

You feel fear when you sense danger. Your heart might race, and your insides might feel shaky. Don't worry! Fear helps protect us.
Are you afraid of anything?

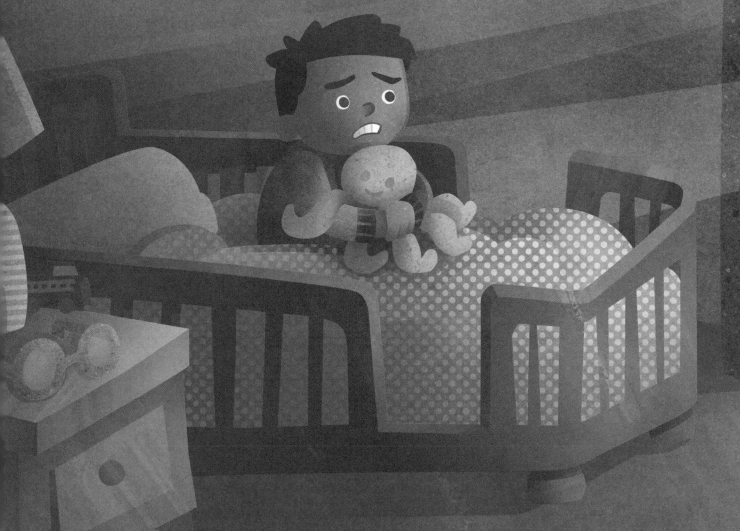

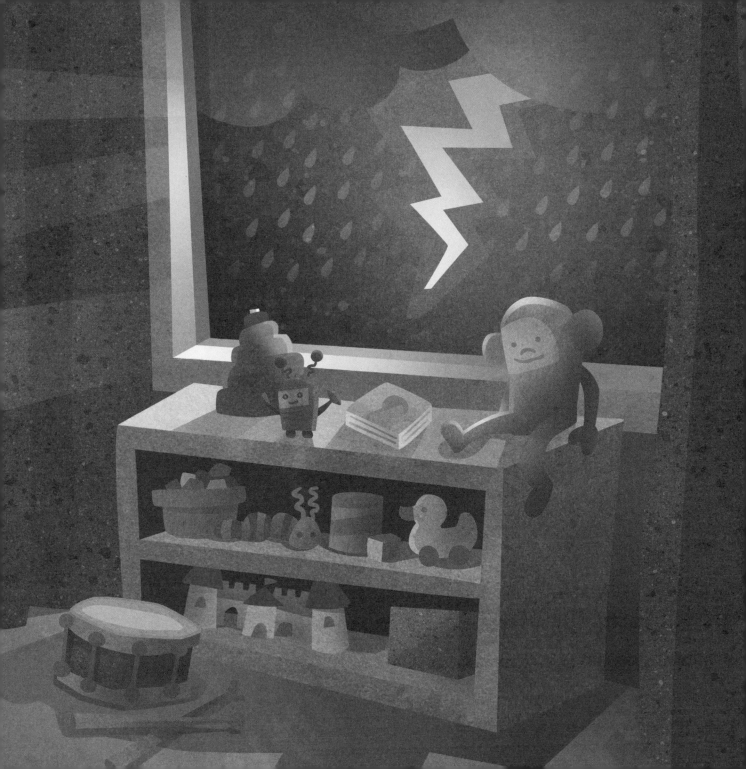

When you are sad, your body feels tired.
Your mouth frowns, and you might cry.
What makes you sad?

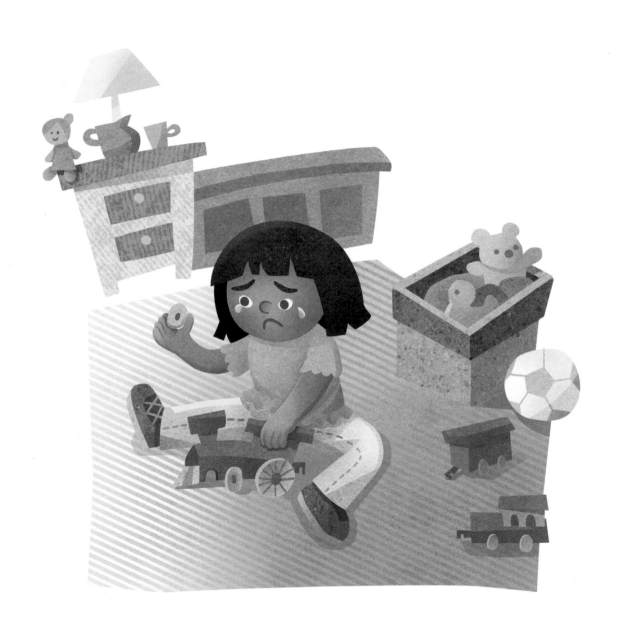

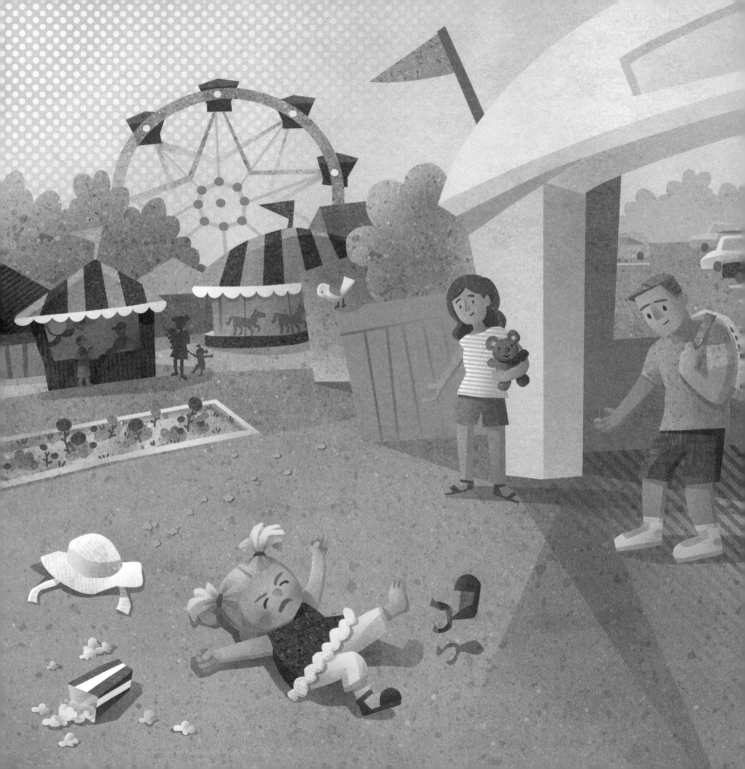

When you are angry, your insides
might feel hot and bubbly.
You might clench your fists and shout, "No!"
Have you ever been angry?

You feel disgust when you find something icky. You might wrinkle your nose and say, "Ewww!" What do you find disgusting?

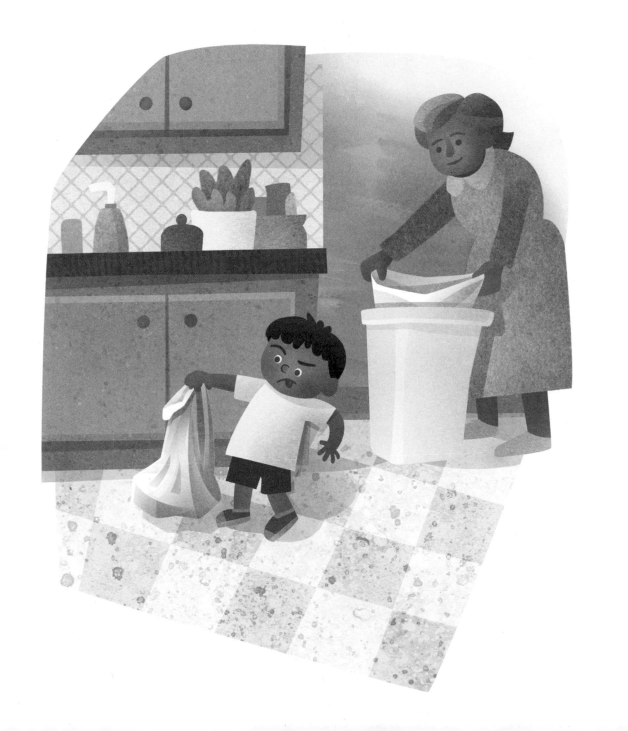

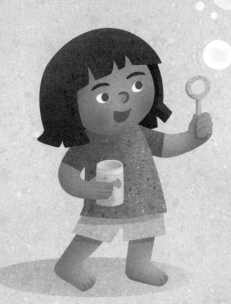

We all feel these emotions.

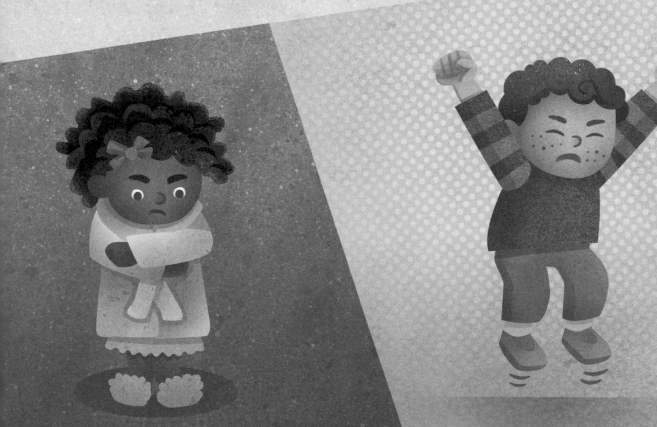

And we all feel them differently.

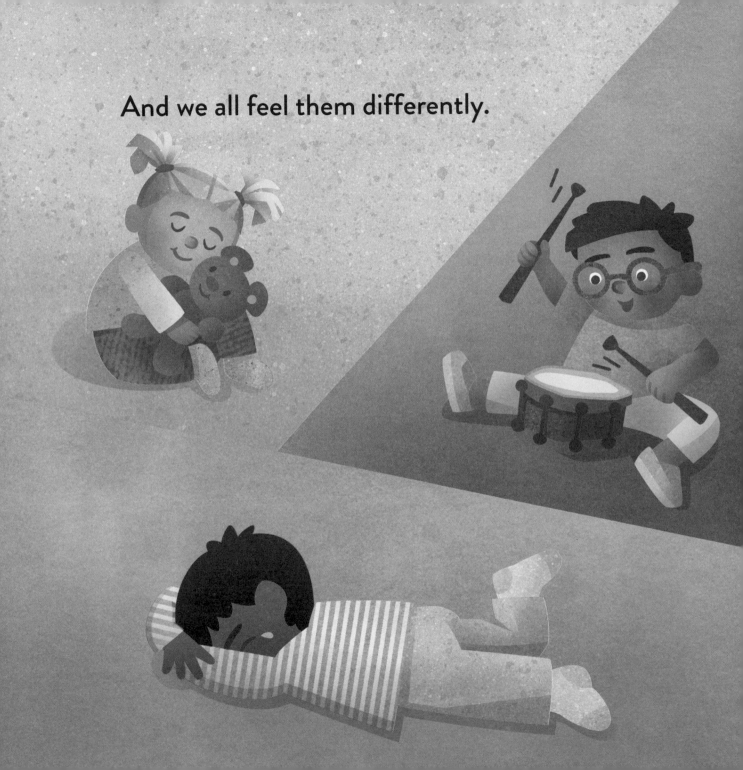

When emotions feel too big, tell a grown-up. They can help you!

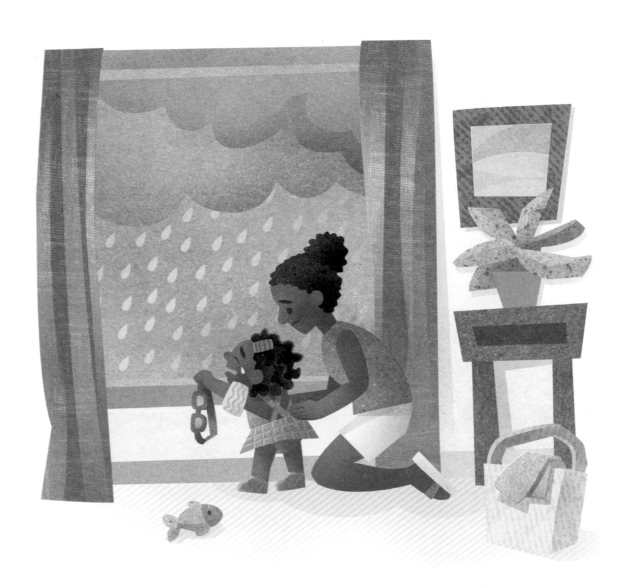

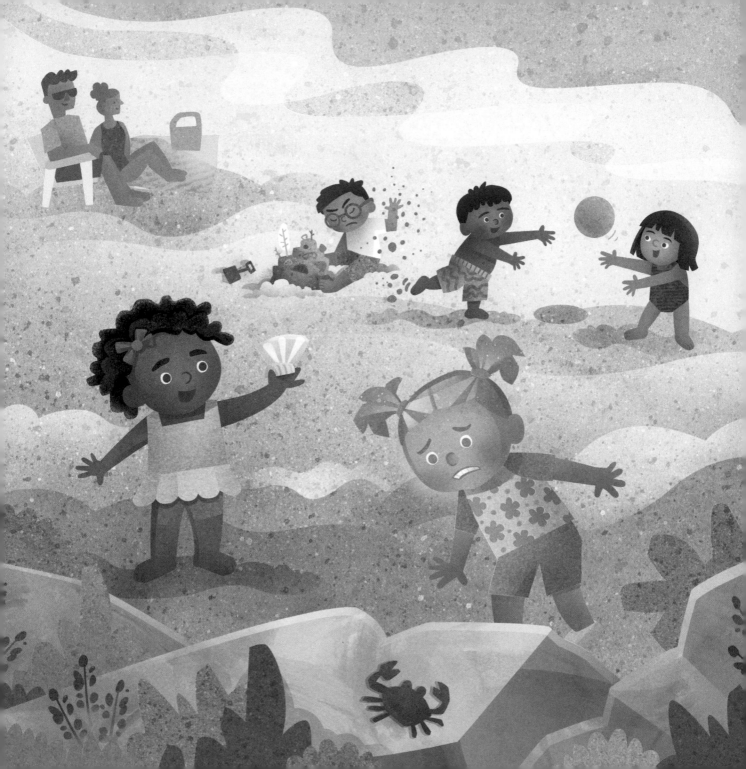

We don't feel happy *all* the time.
Different emotions bring lots of different
thoughts, feelings, and actions.

It's nice feeling happy!
Happiness might make you wiggle or sing.

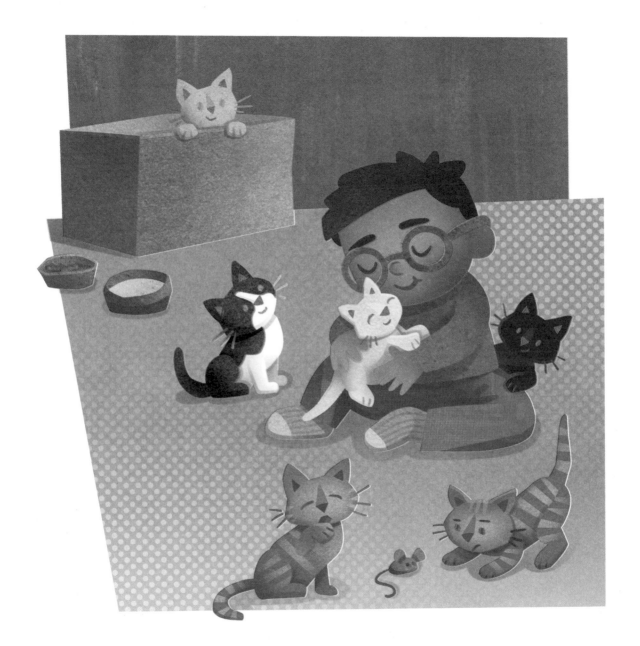

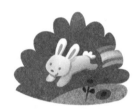

When you feel surprised,
you might jump or yell.

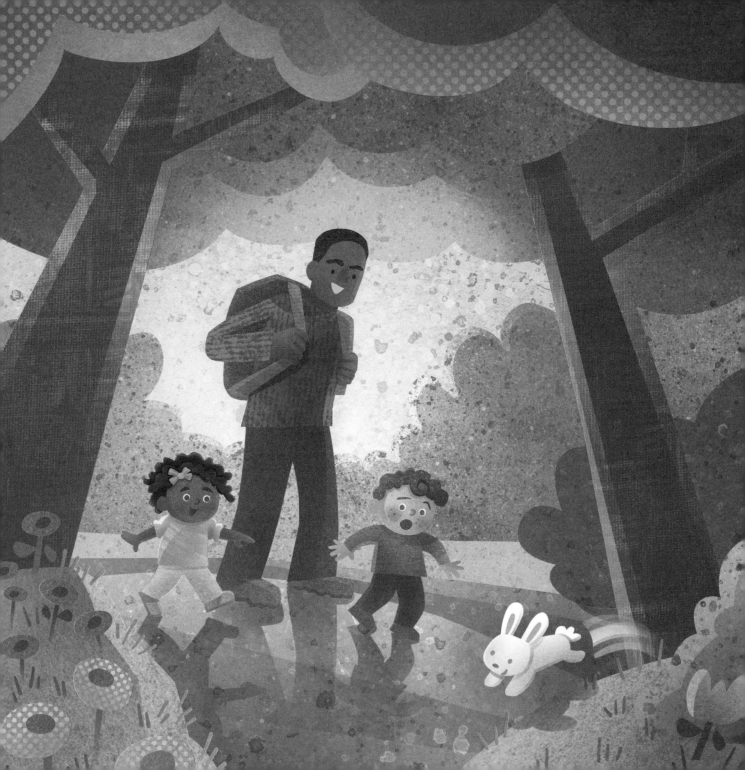

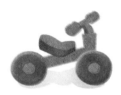

Feeling fear might make you
want to run or hide, and that's okay.
This emotion helps keep you safe.

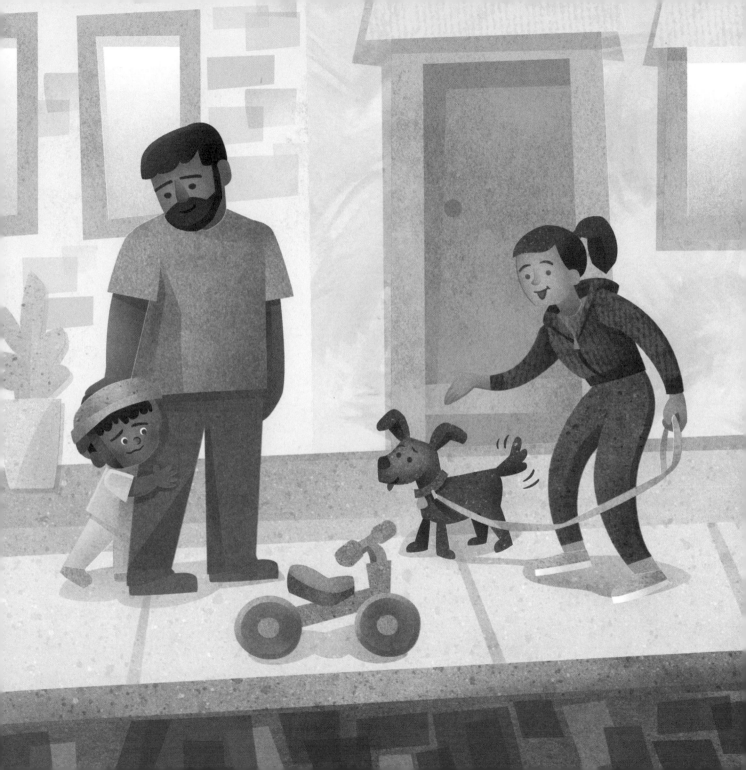

Feeling sad is like when you're not feeling well. Kindness from others can make sadness disappear.

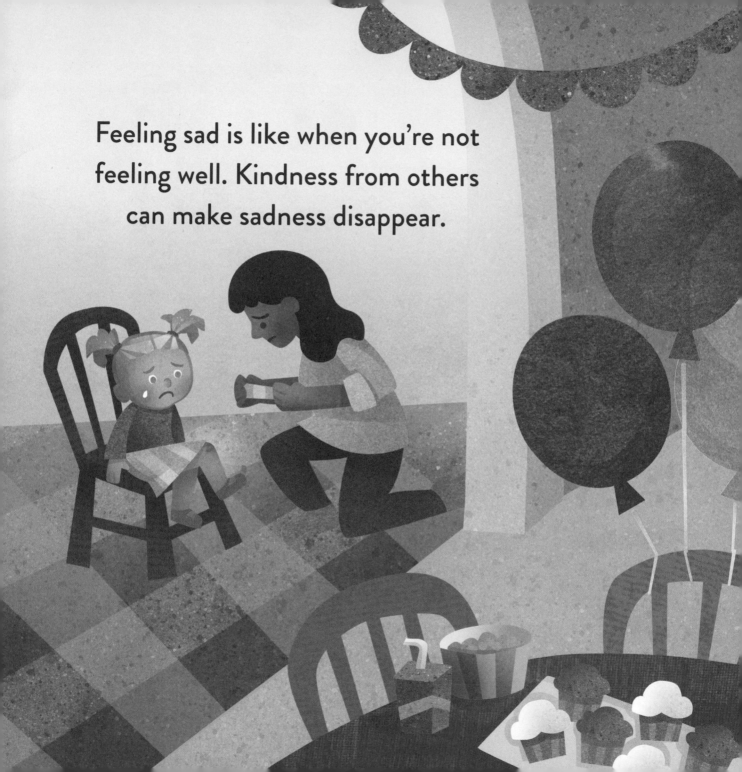

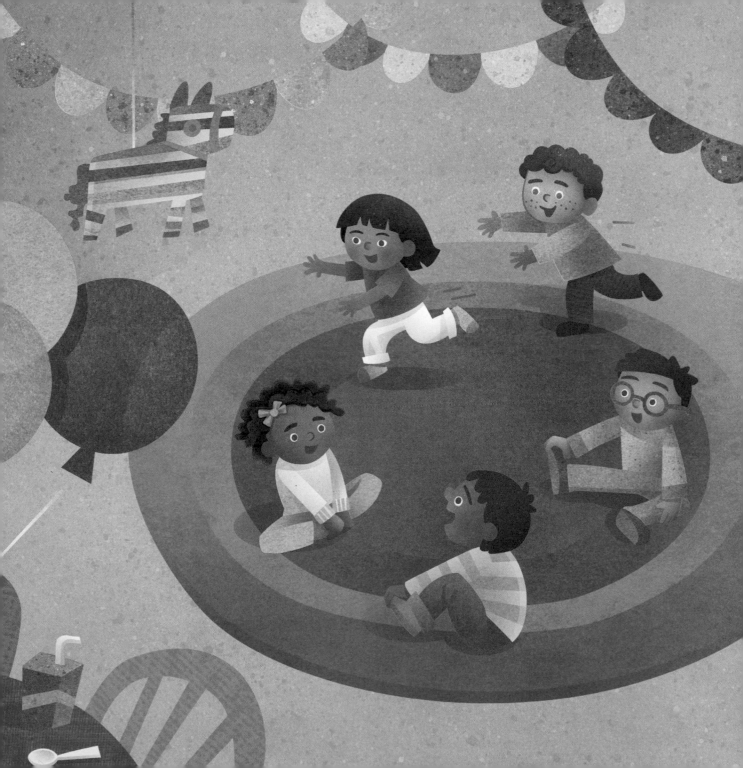

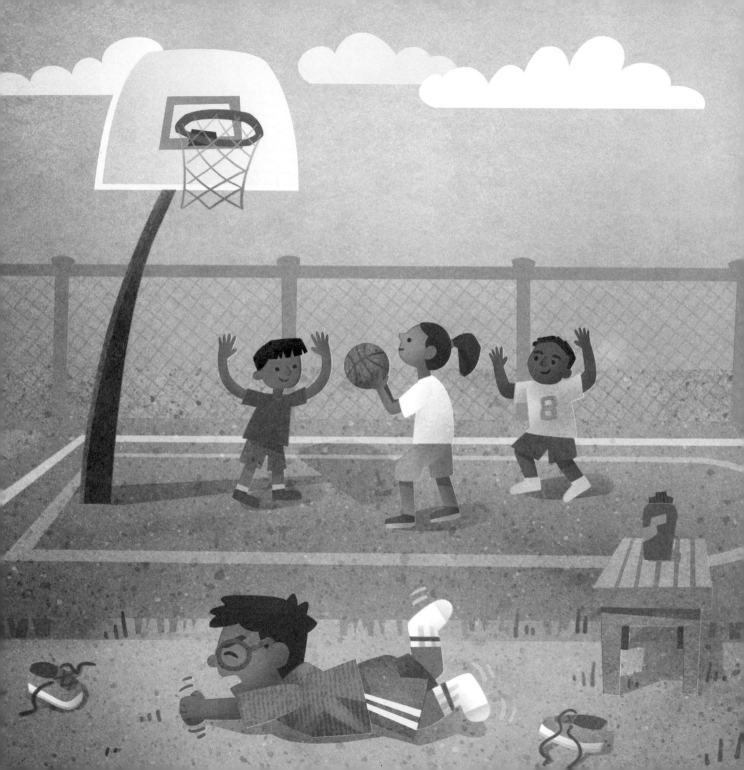

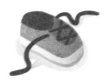

Not getting what you want might make you feel angry. This emotion helps us relieve stress. Instead of getting loud, try talking nicely.

If you're feeling disgust, you might want to turn from or move away from whatever is gross.

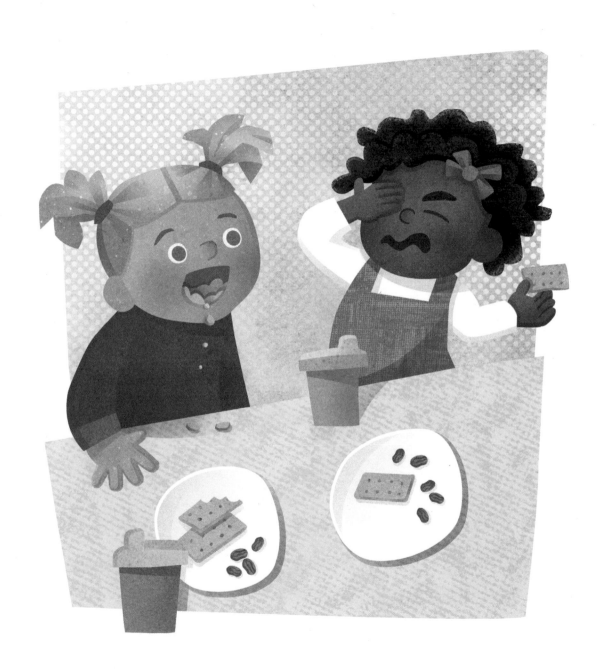

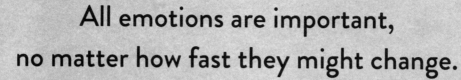

All emotions are important,
no matter how fast they might change.

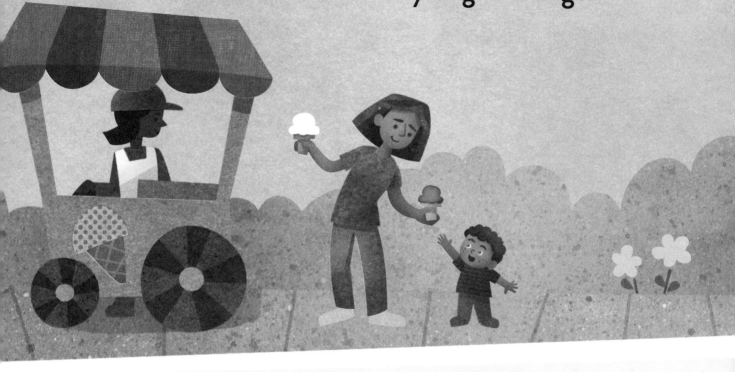

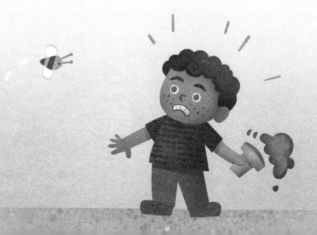

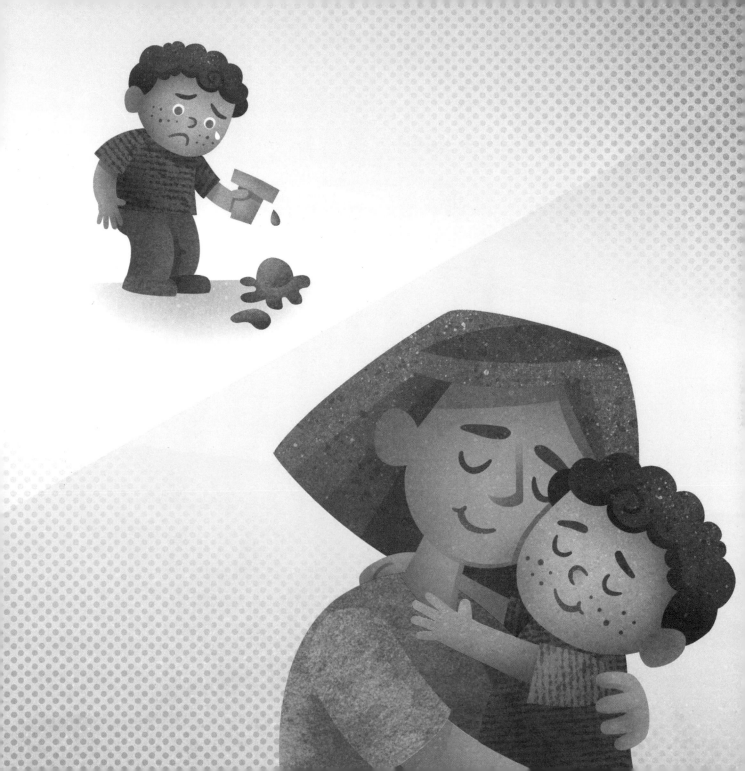

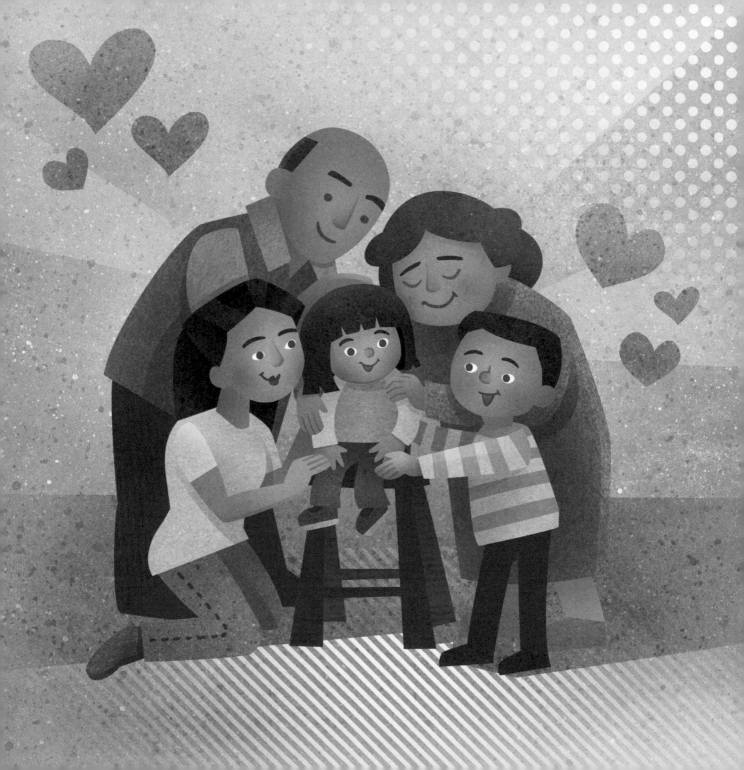

Your emotions are perfect.
Big or small, love them all!

A Note to Grown-Ups

To clarify, emotions are instinctive reactions. Feelings are reactions to emotions. That is, we feel our emotions. Behavior is how we act in response to whatever created an emotion.

As you know, toddlers have big emotions that change quickly. Teaching young children about their emotions and feelings will help both of you manage strong emotions as well as help them develop emotional intelligence as they grow.

Here are some ways to help your little one better understand their own emotions:

1. Regularly express your own emotions verbally. For example, "I enjoy being outside. I feel happy." This will help model for toddlers how they can express their emotions the same way.

2. Help your toddler label their emotions. You could say, "It looks like you're having fun on the swings. Do you feel happy right now?"

3. Help them identify other people's emotions. This could be in real life or books. For example, "The girl in the book has lost her dog. How do you think she feels?"

4. Teach your children techniques to help them calm down, like slowly breathing deeply, grabbing their blanket, or listening to soothing music. Practice this together even when they're not upset, so when needed, they'll already know what to do.

5. When your toddler is angry, remember to put on your own oxygen mask first. Humans have "mirror neurons," so it's normal to feel the same emotion you see being expressed. You can't help them calm down when you're also angry and upset! Kindly (but firmly) set boundaries. For example, if your toddler is upset because they can't have a cookie, they shouldn't get a cookie just because they scream. Instead, you can empathize by saying something like "I see you're really upset and you'd really like a cookie. You can have another cookie tomorrow after lunch." No further negotiation.

About the Author

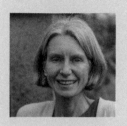 **ORLENA KEREK, MD**, who trained as a pediatric doctor, teaches moms and their families to lead a healthy life in a way that is easy and fun. Check out her podcast *Fit and Fabulous at Forty and Beyond* and her "Road Map to Healthy Amazing You" worksheet on DrOrlena.com.

About the Illustrator

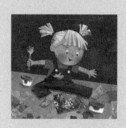 As a little girl, illustrator **APRIL HARTMANN** was very happy whenever she was drawing or painting. In 1993, she earned her BFA in Illustration at the College for Creative Studies in Detroit. Her artwork is now featured in kids' magazines, on toys and packaging, and she has illustrated many books for children. *The Dream Keepers* is her first book as a published author. You can see more of her illustrations on Instagram at @aprilhartmanncreations and her website at AHCreations.com.